YOUR KNOWLEDGE HAS VALUE

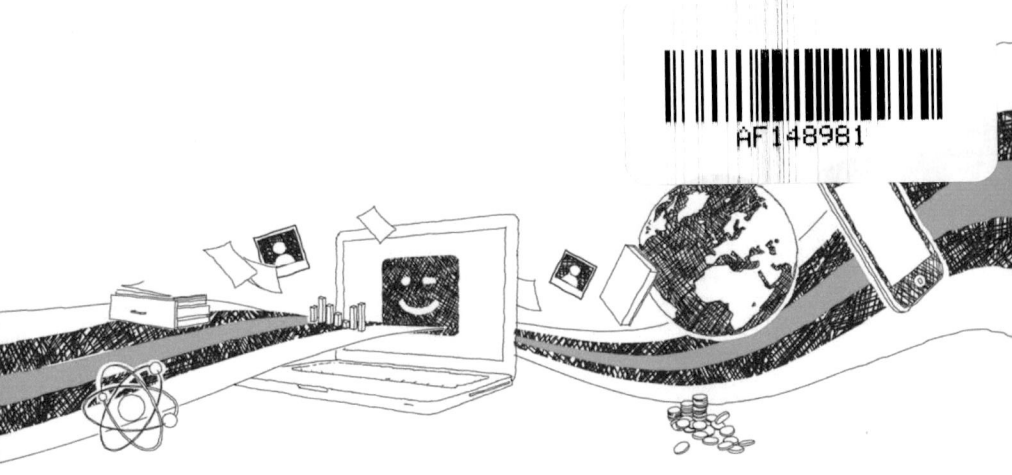

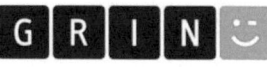

Carol Benjamin

Assessment of Causation in Epidemiologic Research

GRIN Publishing

Bibliographic information published by the German National Library:

The German National Library lists this publication in the National Bibliography; detailed bibliographic data are available on the Internet at http://dnb.dnb.de .

Imprint:

Copyright © 2009 GRIN Verlag GmbH
Print and binding: Books on Demand GmbH, Norderstedt Germany
ISBN: 978-3-656-55127-0

This book at GRIN:

http://www.grin.com/en/e-book/265470/assessment-of-causation-in-epidemiologic-research

GRIN - Your knowledge has value

Since its foundation in 1998, GRIN has specialized in publishing academic texts by students, college teachers and other academics as e-book and printed book. The website www.grin.com is an ideal platform for presenting term papers, final papers, scientific essays, dissertations and specialist books.

Visit us on the internet:

http://www.grin.com/

http://www.facebook.com/grincom

http://www.twitter.com/grin_com

Assessment of Causation in Epidemiologic Research

Carol Benjamin

TUI University

Abstract

In this assignment I assessed the relationship between soy consumption and breast cancer which has been studied by Sacks et al (2006), Messina & Loprinzi (2001), Wu et al (2008), and Trock et al (2006). I used the Bradford Hill criteria and assess whether soy has an inverse causal relationship with breast cancer.

In the article on "Emerging Themes in Epidemiology" Hoffler (2005) explained that Sir Austin Bradford (1897-1991), who was an outstanding pioneer in medical statistics and epidemiology wrote a paper entitled, "The environment and disease: Association or causation" which had an enormous impact on epidemiologists and medical researchers. Hill provided nine considerations for assessing whether an observed association involved a causal component or not. The relationship between soy consumption and breast cancer will be assessed using the Bradford Hill criteria shown below.

1. Strength of Association

This association is related to the relative risk and odds ratio whereby there can be a weak, moderate or strong association. Article by Trock et al. (2006) proposed that high intake of soy foods has been proposed to contribute to the low breast cancer risk in Asian countries. However, results of epidemiologic studies of this association are highly variable, and experimental data suggest that soy constituents can be estrogenic and potentially risk enhancing. A meta-analysis of 18 epidemiologic studies was completed and examined soy exposure and breast cancer risk. The authors demonstrated that in a pooled analysis, among all women, high soy intake was modestly associated with reduced breast cancer risk. Odds ratio =0.86, 95% confidence interval = 0.75 to 0.99. The association was not statistically significant among women in Asian countries. The Odds Ratio =0.89, 95% confidence interval = 0.71 to 1.12. Trock and his colleagues argue that among the 10 studies that stratified by menopausal status the inverse association between soy exposure and breast cancer risk was somewhat stronger in premenopausal women. Odds Ratio = 0.70, 95% confidence interval = 0.58 to 0.85) than in post menopausal women. Odds ratio = 0.77, 95% confidence interval – 0.60 to 0.98. Trock and colleague concluded that soy intake may be associated with a small reduction in breast cancer risk.

2. Consistency of Association

Weed (2000) explained consistency as the extent to which the association is observed in different circumstances, by different investigators, using different study design and in different locations. The relationship between soy consumption is consistent among a large number of studies. From the studies that I reviewed they all showed that there is a relationship between soy exposure and breast cancer. Messina and Loprinzi's (2001) article was written to highlight studies that pertain mostly to the controversy of the relationship to soy exposure and breast cancer. Although Weed reviewed many studies that reveal a relationship between soy exposure and breast cancer, I will only mention a few of the studies in this assignment. The author explains that several studies examined the effects of different soy products on the development of chemically induced mammary cancer in adult animals. The data are somewhat inconsistent but generally show that in comparison with control diets, the substitution of soy protein for other protein typically found in a standard laboratory diet modestly reduced (25-50%) tumor incidence. Weed mentioned studies that were completed by Barnes et al. (1990), Hakkak et al (2000) and Ohta et al. (2000). Weed also reviewed studies completed by Cohen et al. (2000) and Hsueh (1992) which argued that soy did not show protective effects on breast cancer.

Weed concluded that there is a lack of any convincing information to substantiate either of two extreme and opposing claims which states that soy is protective against breast cancer and that soy is harmful for women with a history of or at high risk for breast cancer. Although the article shows that there are opposing views, all the articles that were

4

reviewed showed that there is a relationship between soy exposure and breast cancer. As a result there is a consistency of relations.

3. Specificity of Association

Article by Sacks et al. (2006) shows that soy protein has gained considerable attention for their potential in improving risk factors for cardiovascular disease. In the randomized trials, isolated soy protein with isoflavones, as compared with milk or other protein, decreased LDL cholesterol concentration and the average effect was 3%. The author argued that this reduction is very is very small relative to the large amount of protein tested in the studies. There were no significant effects on HDL cholesterol, triglycerides, lipoprotein or blood pressure.

4. Temporality Relationship

Many studies reveal that soy consumption will precede breast cancer outcome. Many cohort studies reviewed provide convincing evidence for temporality since they are less likely to have been affected by information bias. An article titled "Soy Food Intake Associated with Better Breast Cancer Outcomes" shows that breast cancer recurrence and overall mortality are lower among women who eat soy foods after their initial diagnosis. This article reveals that five thousands survivors of breast cancer in Shanghai provided information on lifestyle six months after their diagnosis and during several subsequent interviews. After a median four years' follow-up, women in the highest quartile of soy consumption (for example, tofu, soy milk, or fresh soy beans) showed lower hazard ratios for total mortality and recurrence, relative to those in the lowest quartile. This confirms that soy consumption precede breast cancer outcome.

5. Dose Response (Biological Gradient)

Many studies have shown that the amount of soy intake is associated with protection against breast cancer. Wu et al. (2006) article explained that meta-analysis of eight studies conducted in high soy consuming Asians show a significant trend of decreasing risk with increasing soy food intake. The studies show that compared to the lowest level of soy food intake (< 5 mg isoflavones per day), risk was intermediate (odds ratio = 0.88, 95% confidence interval = 0.78 – 0.98). Among those with modest risk (~ 10 mg isoflavones per day) intake and lowest (odds ratio = 0.71, 95 % confidence interval =0.60 – 0.85) among those with high intake (> 20 mg isoflavones per day). Wu stated that in contrast, soy intake was unrelated to breast cancer risk in studies conducted in the eleven low soy consuming Western populations whose average highest and lowest soy isoflavone intake levels were around 0.8 and 0.15 mg per day. The authors argue that the evidence that is based on case-control studies suggest that soy food intake in the amount consumed in Asian populations may have protective effects against breast cancer.

6. Biological Plausibility

Weed explained (2000) explained this criterion as the extent to which an observed association in epidemiological studies is supported or not by the mechanism of action and the underlying disease. An article on Mammographic Density revealed that the American Association for Cancer Research has illustrated new research on Mammographic density. This article argued that women who have a decrease in breast density over a six-year period may have a decreased risk of developing breast cancer compared with women whose breast density remained stable. In this study there is no mention of the relationship between breast cancer and soy exposure.

7. Coherence

In Brandon Hill-Criteria, Coherence is similar to biological Plausibility.

8. Experiment Evidence

In experimental evidence causation is more likely if evidence is based on random assignment with two different groups. Messina and Loprinzi article argued that it is difficult to summarize the surprisingly large numbers of studies that have recently examined the effects of soy consumption on hormonal patterns because of the different experimental designs, number of measures taken and conflicting results. One study has been responsible for raising concerns about soy consumption by breast cancer patients. Messina and colleague reviewed Petrakis et al. (1996) research and found that daily soy consumption over five months was associated with an increase in breast nipple aspirate fluid secretion and breast cell hyperplasia in premenopausal women. Previous epidemiologic research showed that non lactating women who can secrete breast fluid are at an increased breast cancer risk compare to those who cannot.

9. Analogy

The analogy criterion is the least important of all the criteria and will not be addressed in this assignment.

Conclusion

The results of the various studies that were mentioned in this assignment, show that soy consumption has an inverse causal relationship with breast cancer. Other studies show that this relationship does not exist. The available data indicate the lack of any convincing information to substantiate either of the two extreme opposing claims. These claims states that soy is protective against breast cancer and soy is harmful for women with a history of or at high risk for breast cancer. Although the studies cannot substantiate either view, there is definitely a causal relationship between soy consumption and breast cancer. By using the Bradford Hill criteria the assessment of the relationship between soy consumption was determined.

Reference

Hoffler, M. (2005). The Bradford Hill considerations on causality: a counterfactual

perspective. Emerging Themes in Epidemiology, 2(11). Retrieved August 11, 2009,

from http://www.ete-online.com/content/2/1/11

Mammographic Density and Breast Cancer Risk. Retrieved May 16, 2010 from:

http://www.medicexchange.com/Mammography/mammographic-density-and-breast-

cancer-risk.html

Messina, M. J. and Loprinzi, C.L (2001). Soy for Breast Cancer Survivors: A Critical

Review of the Literature. American Society for Nutritional Sciences, 131(3095S-

3108S). Retrieved August 11, 2009, from:

http://jn.nutrition.org/cgi/content/full/131/11/3095S

Sacks F.M., Lichtenstein, A., Van Horn, L., Harris, W., Kris-Etherton, P., and Winston,

M. (2006). Soy Protein, Isoflavones, and Cardiovascular Health. Circulation, 98(7).

Retrieved August 11, 2009, from:

http://circ.ahajournals.org/cgi/content/full/113/7/1034

Soy Food Intake Associated with Better Breast Cancer Outcomes. Retrieved May 16,

2010 from: http://firstwatch.jwatch.org/cgi/content/full/2009/1209/2

Trock, B.J., Hilakivi-Clarke, L., Clarke, R. (2006). Meta analysis of soy intake and

breast cancer risk. Journal of the National Cancer Institute, 98(7). Retrieved August

11, 2009, from http://proquest.umi.com/pqdweb

Weed, D.L. (2000). Interpreting epidemiological evidence: how meta-analysis and causal

inference methods are related. International Journal of Epidemiology, 29(387-390).

Retrieved August 11, 2009, from

http://ije.oxfordjournals.org/cgi/content/full/29/3/387

Bradford hill criteria

Wu, A.H., Yu, M.C, Tseng, C-C., Pike, M.C. (2006). Epidemiology of soy exposures

and breast cancer risk. British Journal of Cancer, 98(9-14). Retrieved August 11,

2009, from http://www.nature.com/bjc/journal/v98/n1/full/6604145a.html